Martin goes into hospital

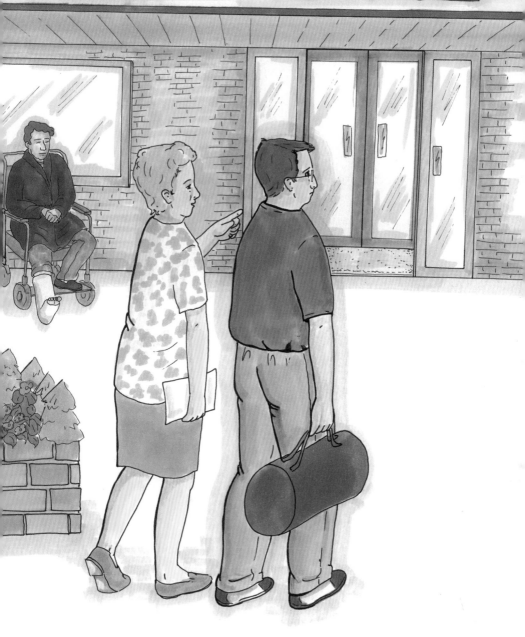

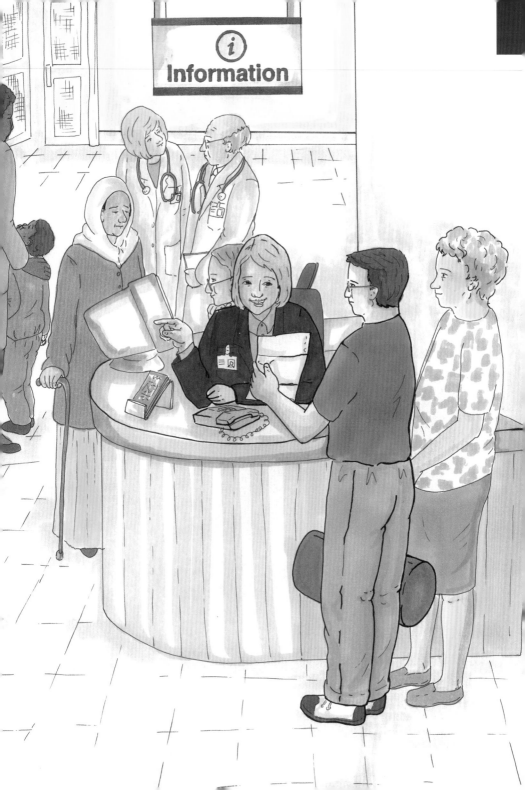

3

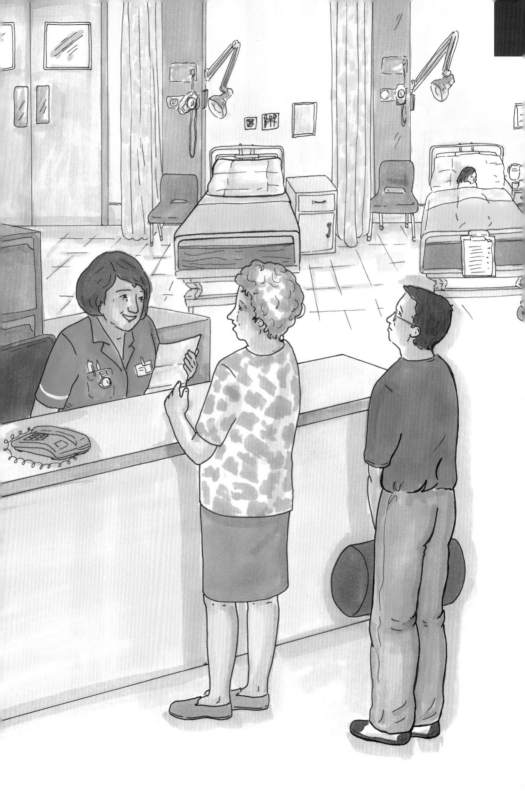

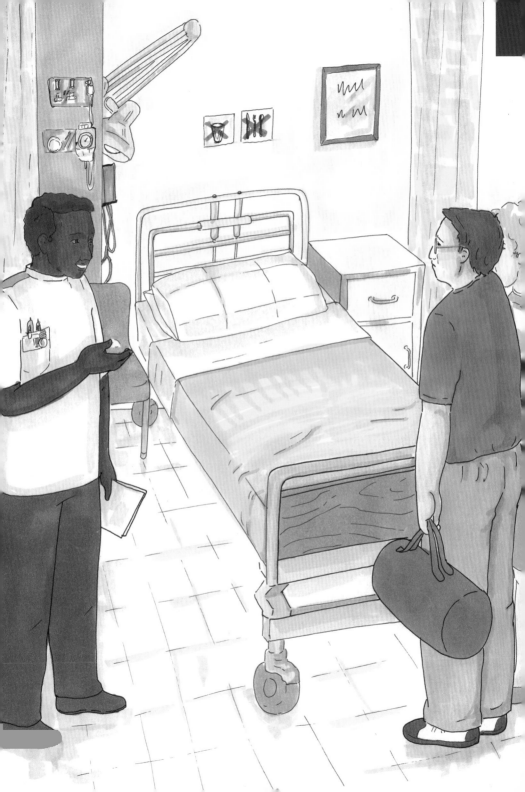

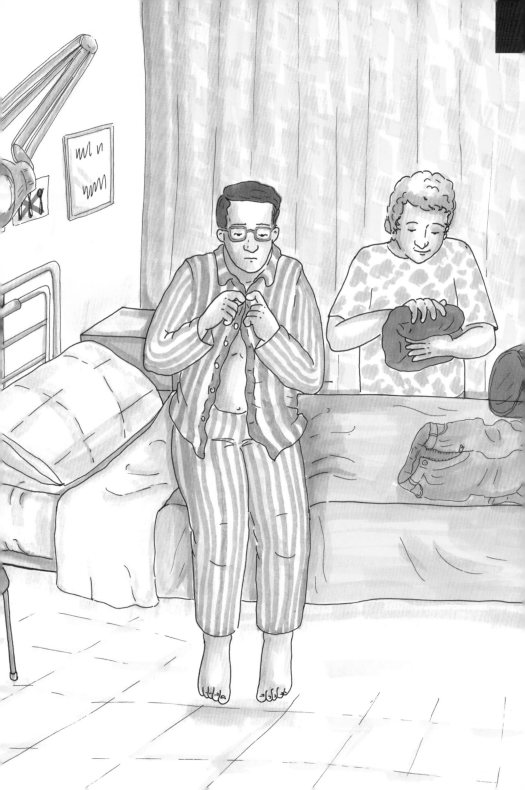

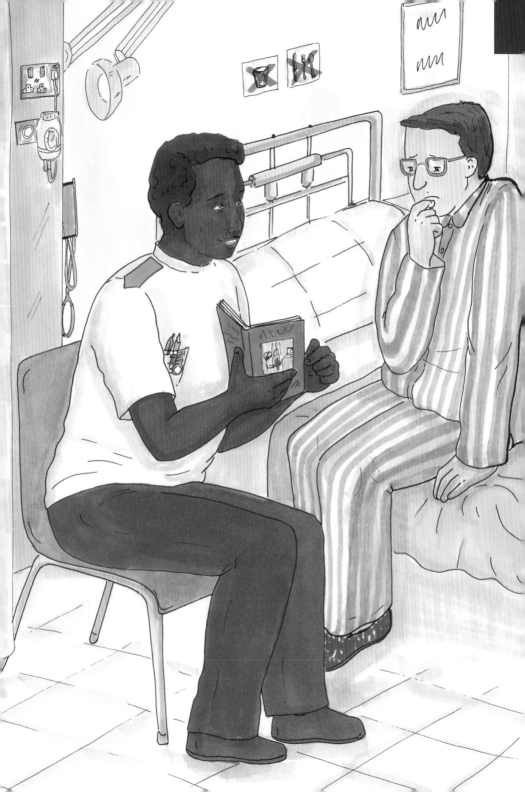

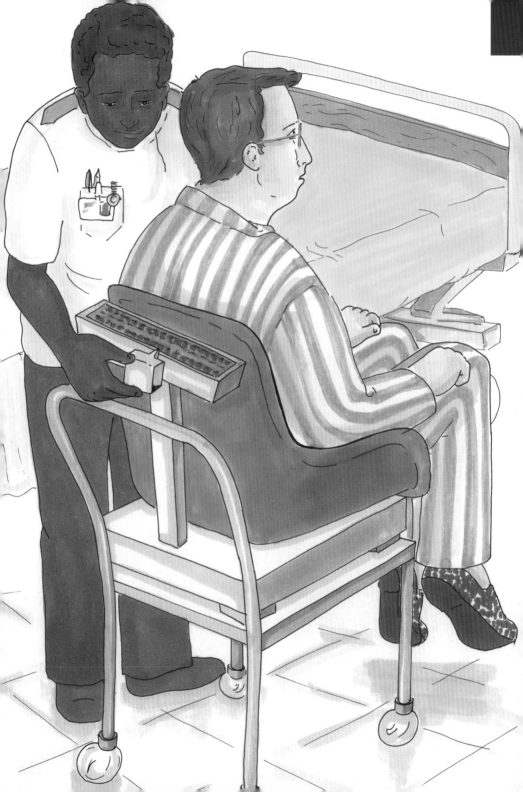

8

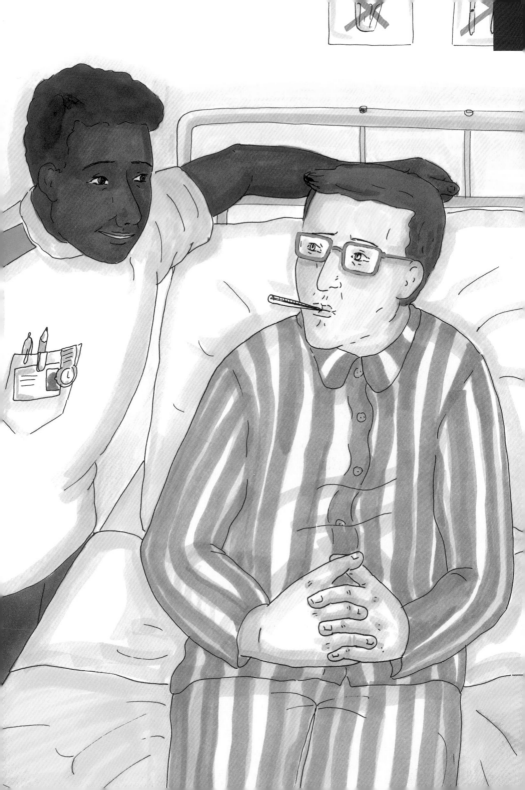

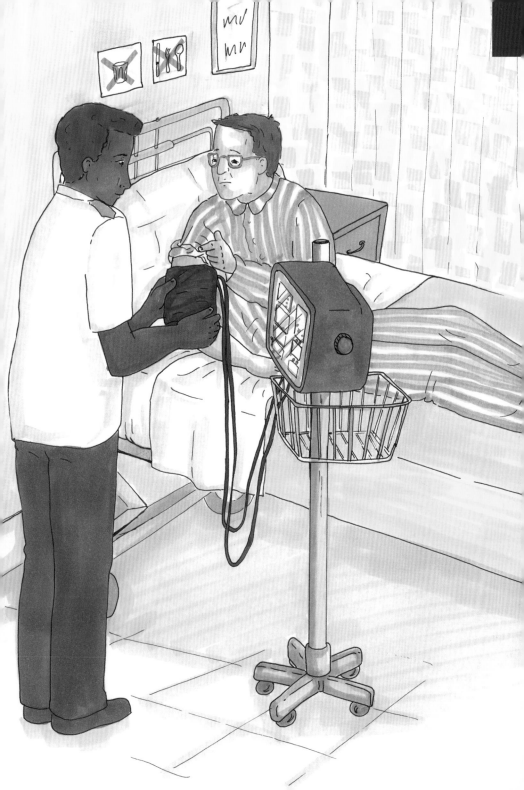

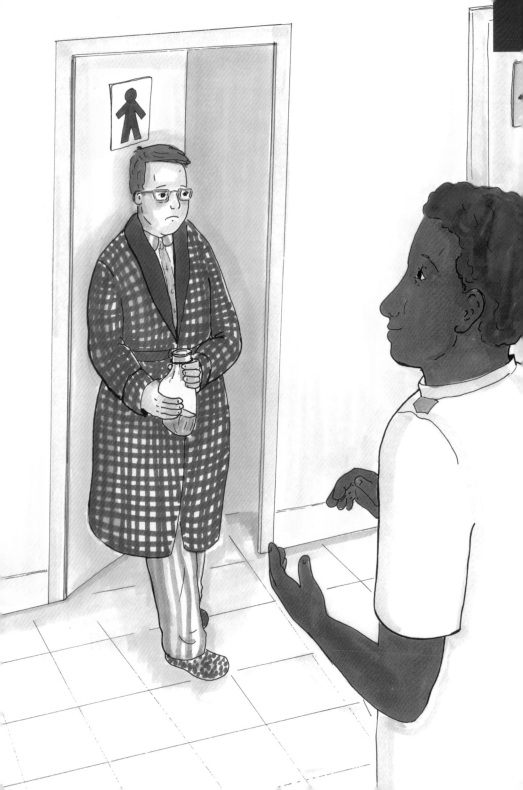

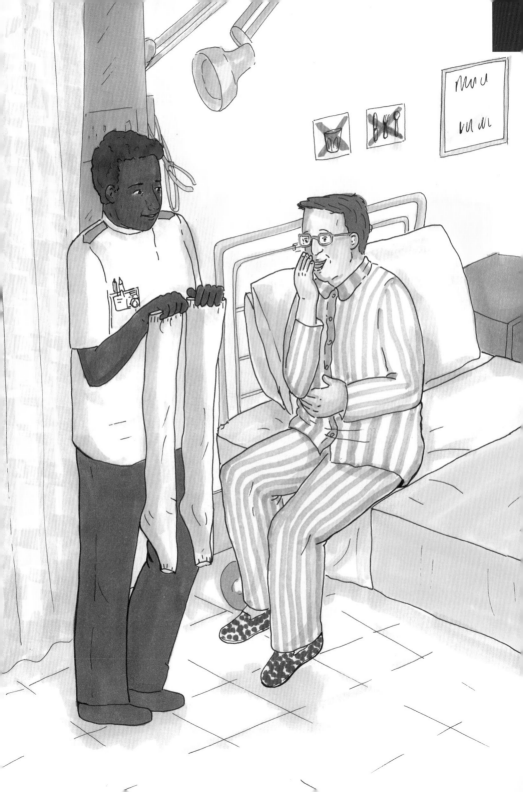

12

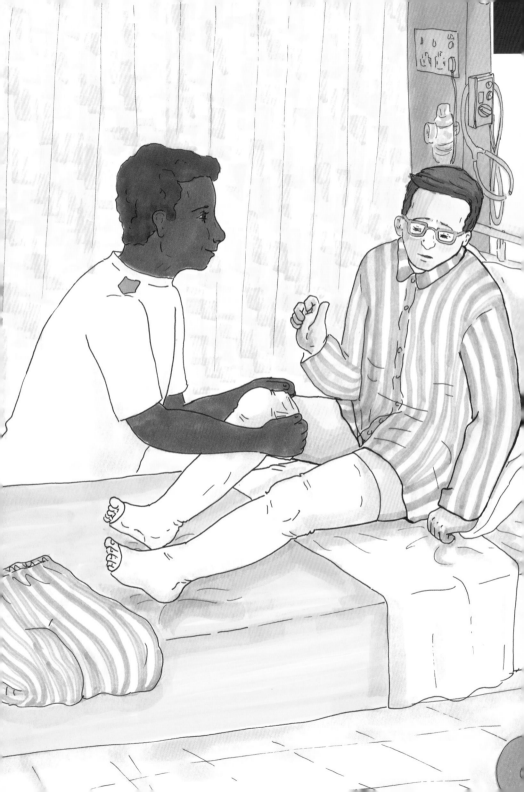

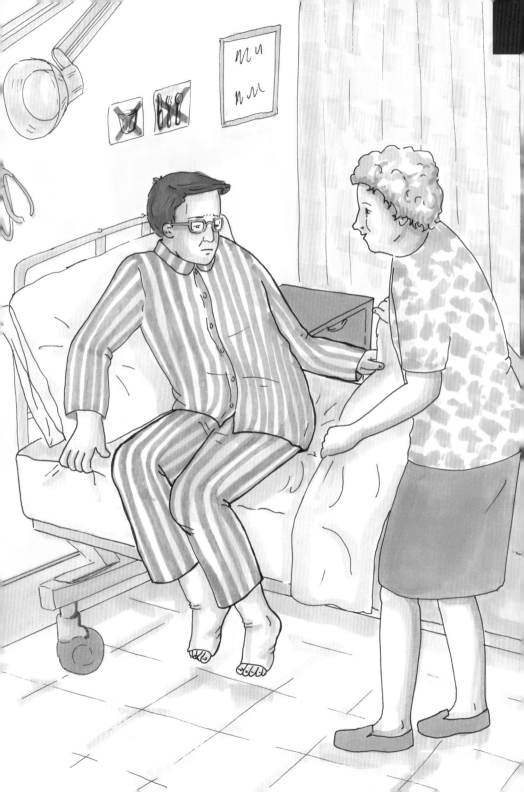

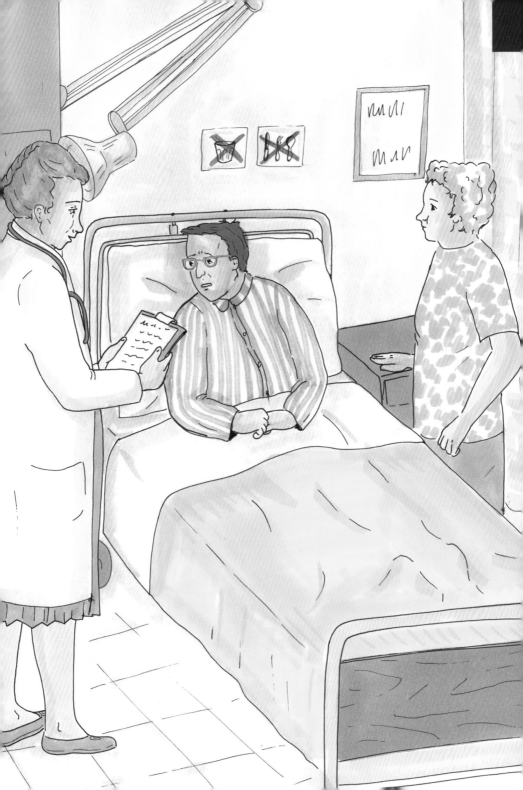

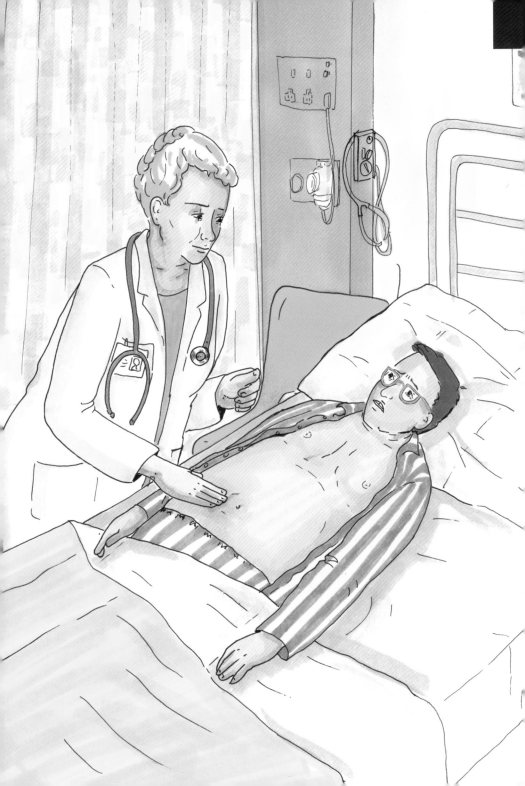

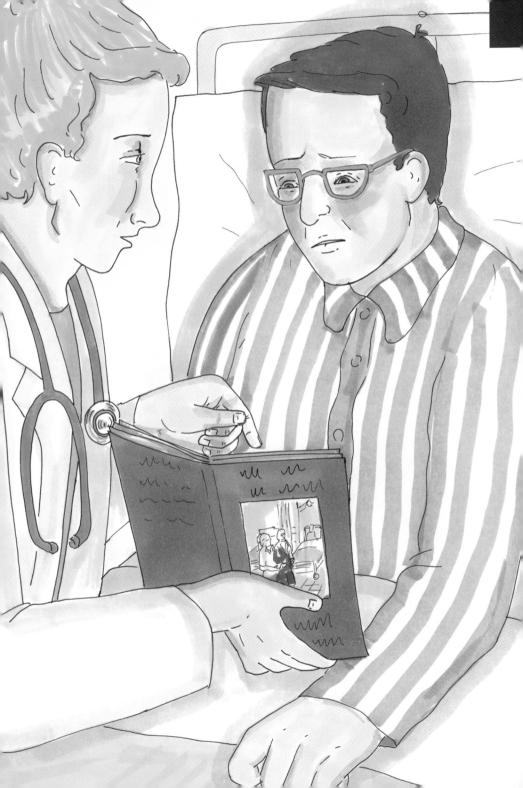

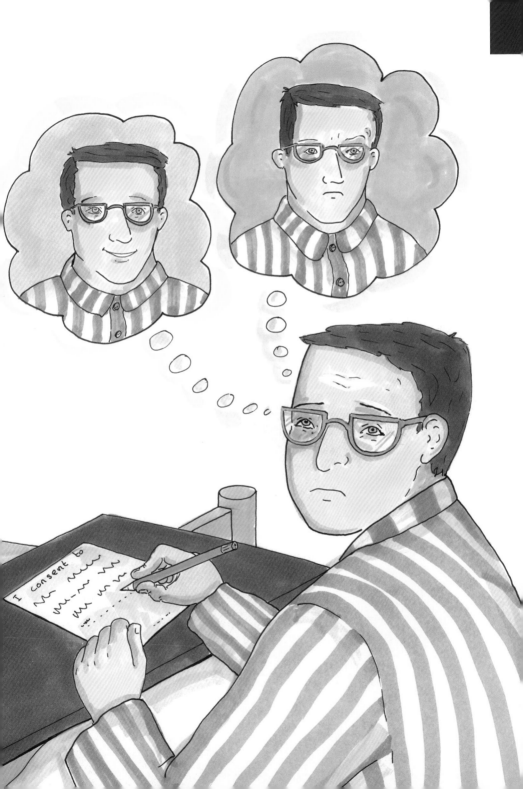

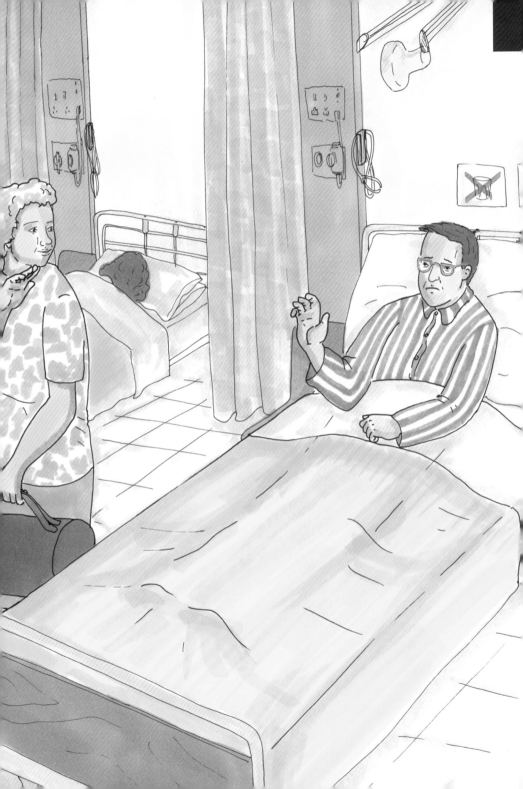

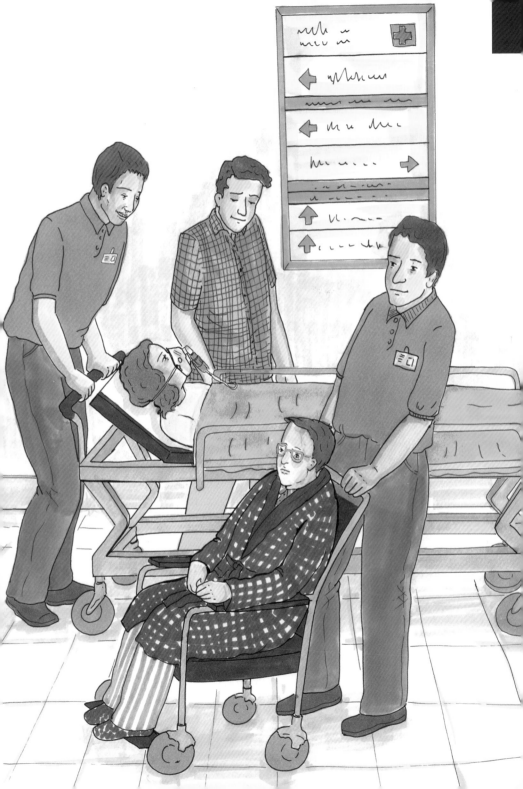

20

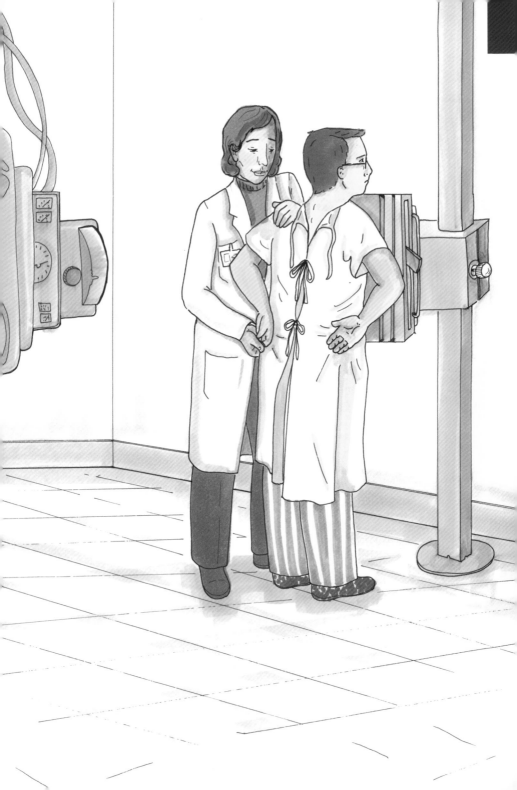

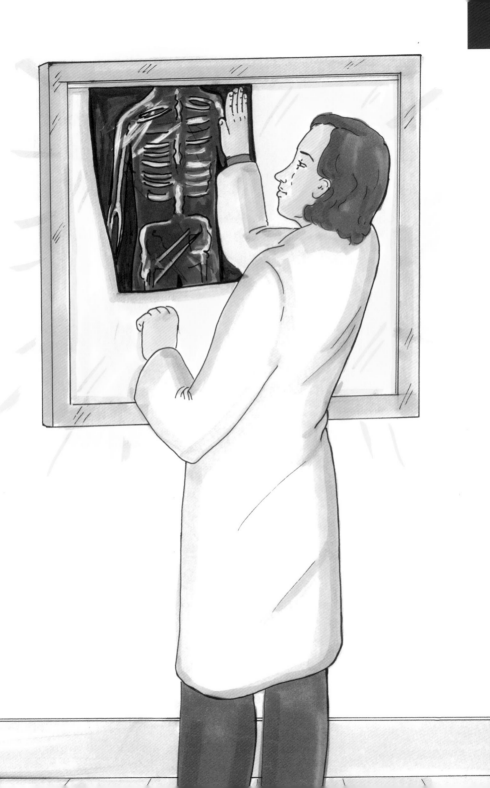

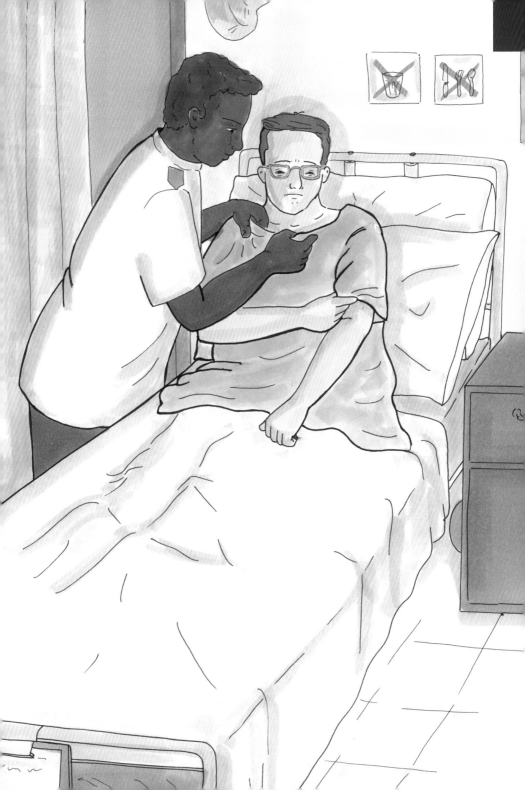

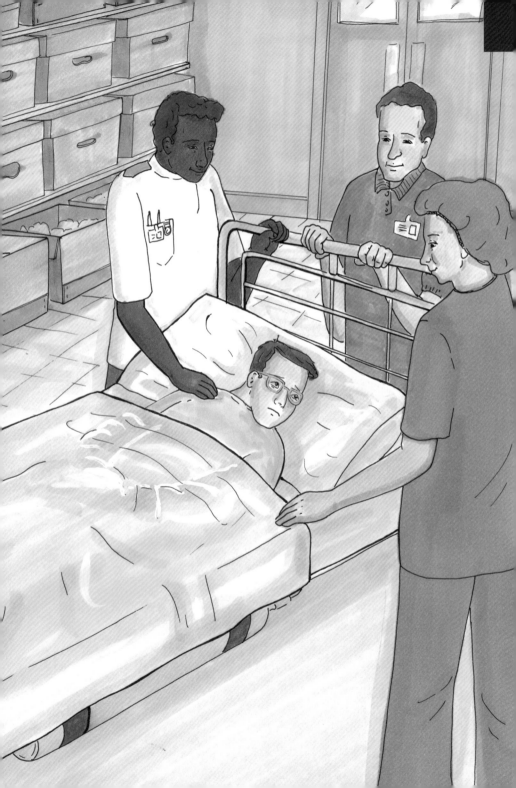

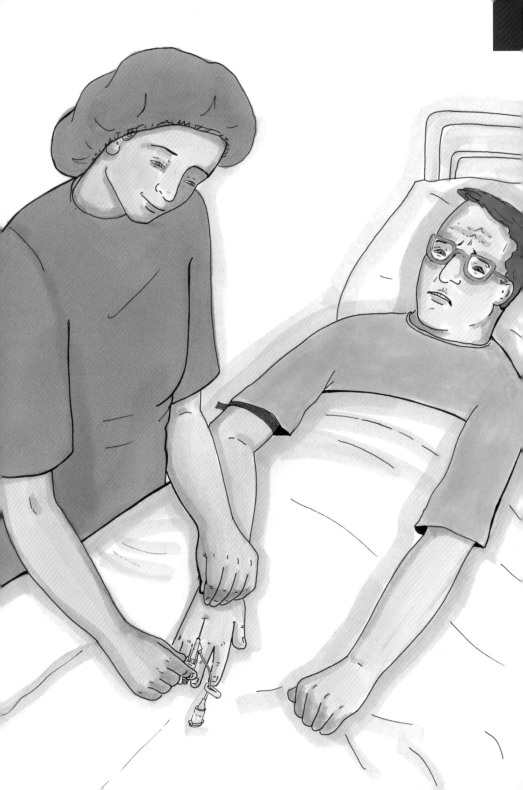

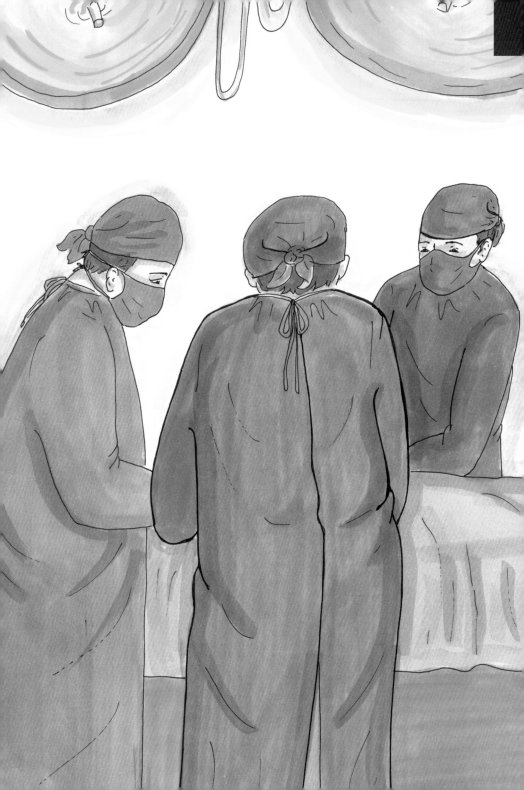

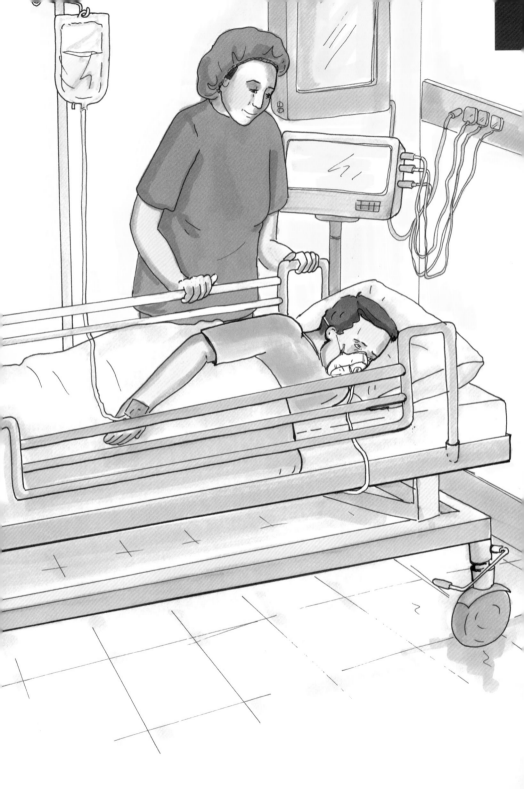

27

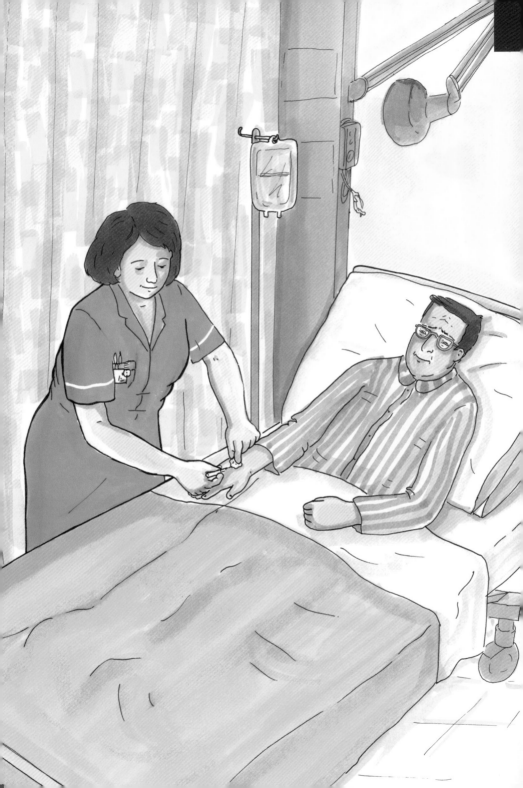

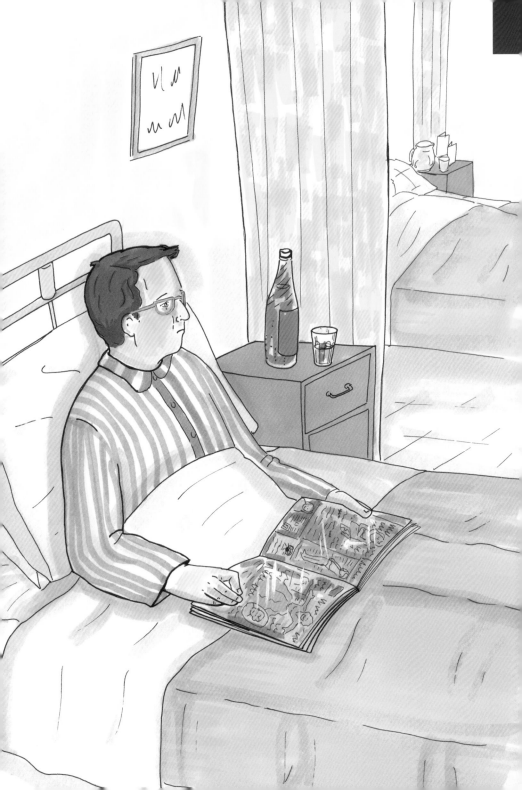

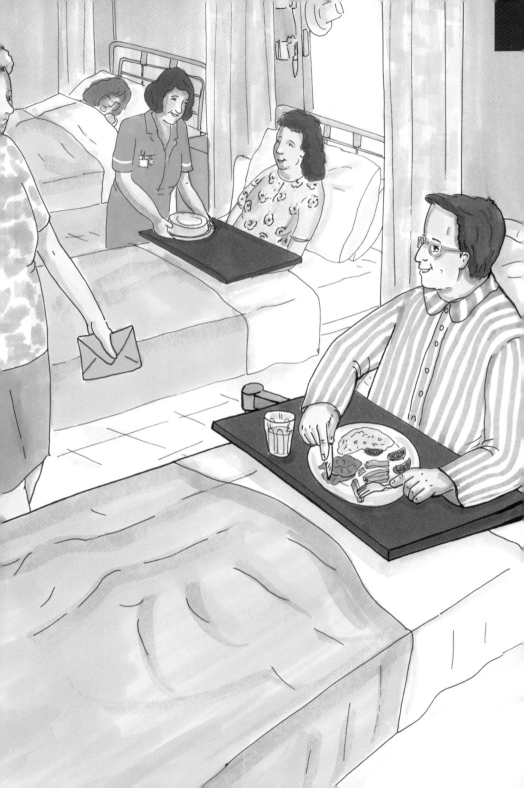

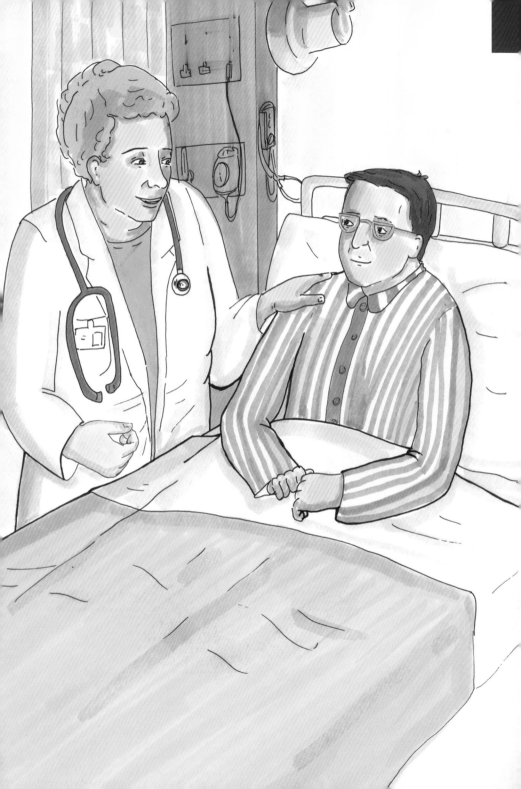

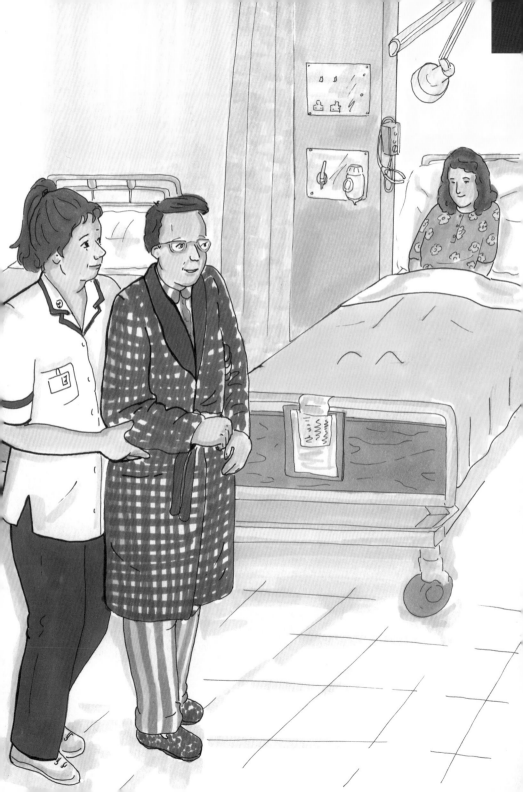

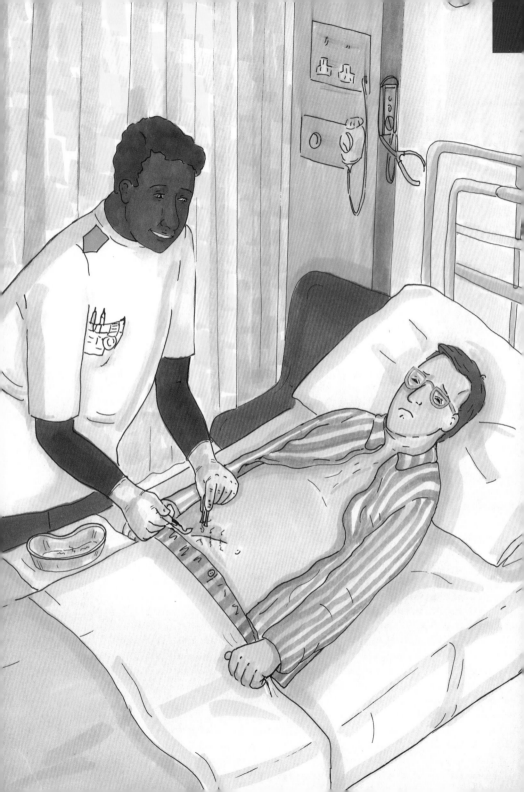

33

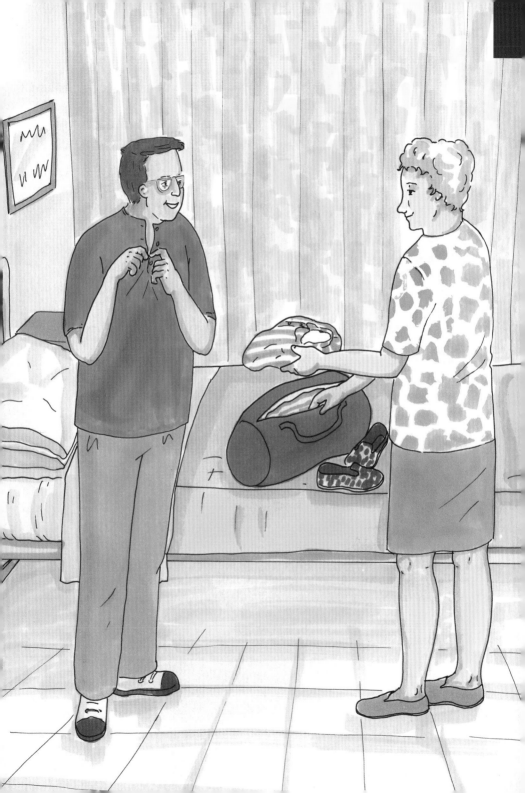

Mary is taken to the emergency department

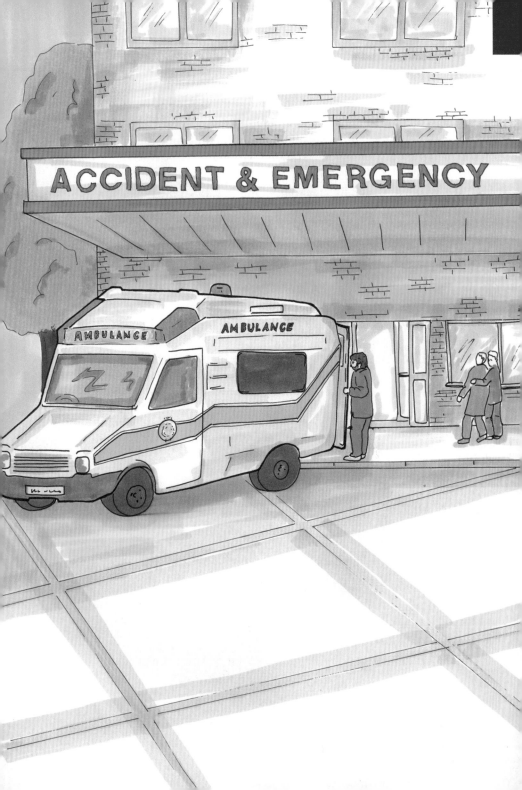

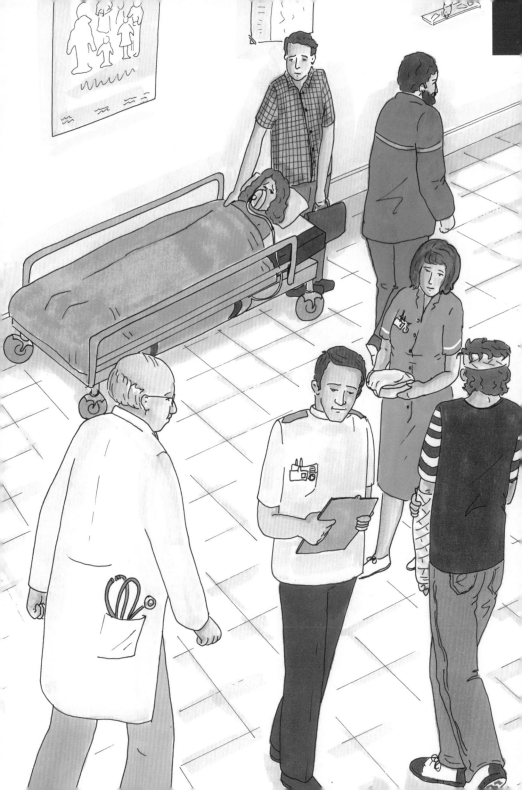

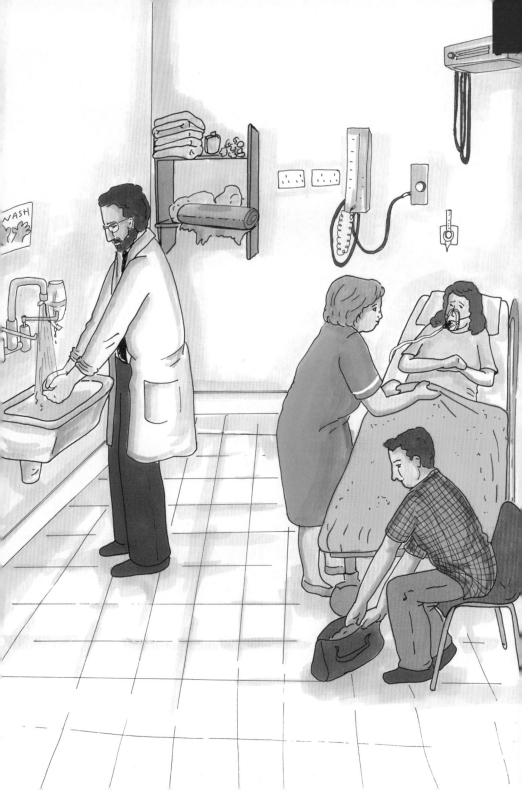

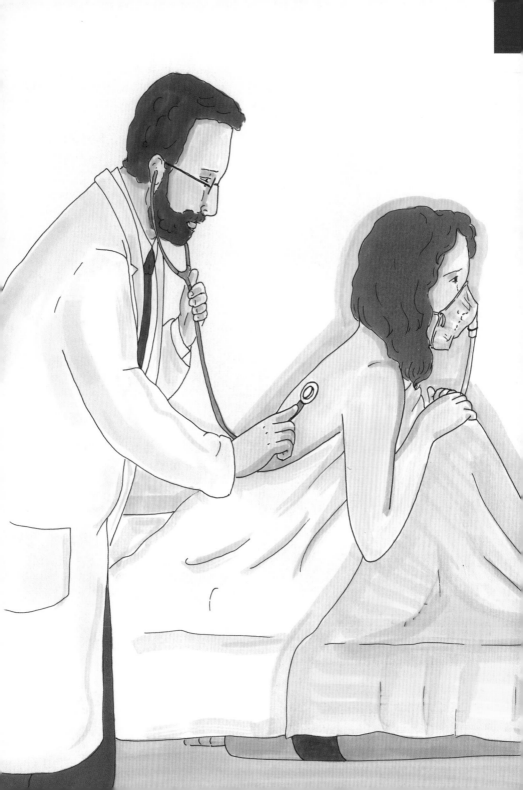

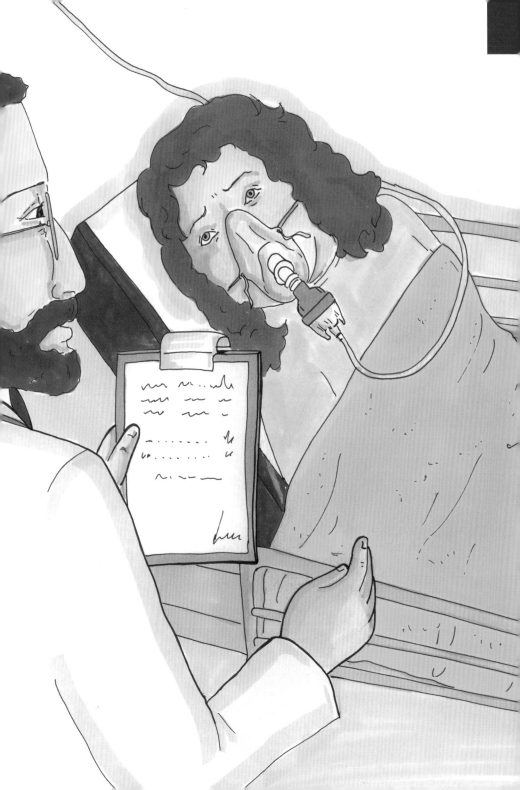

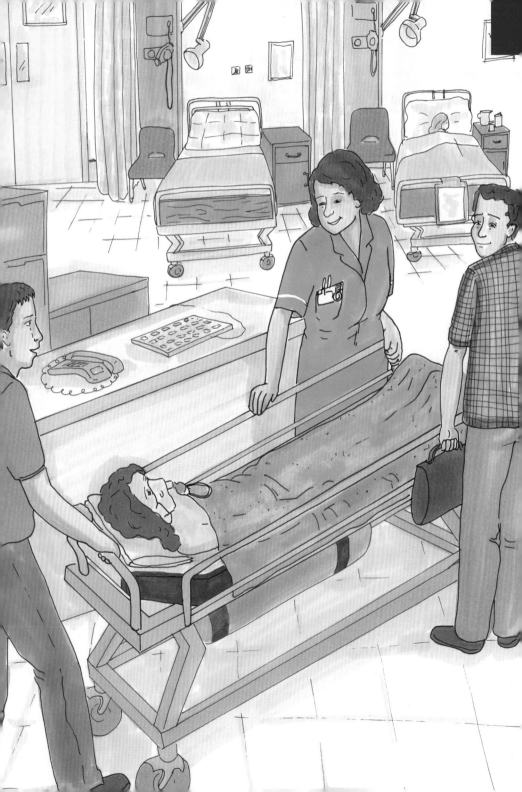

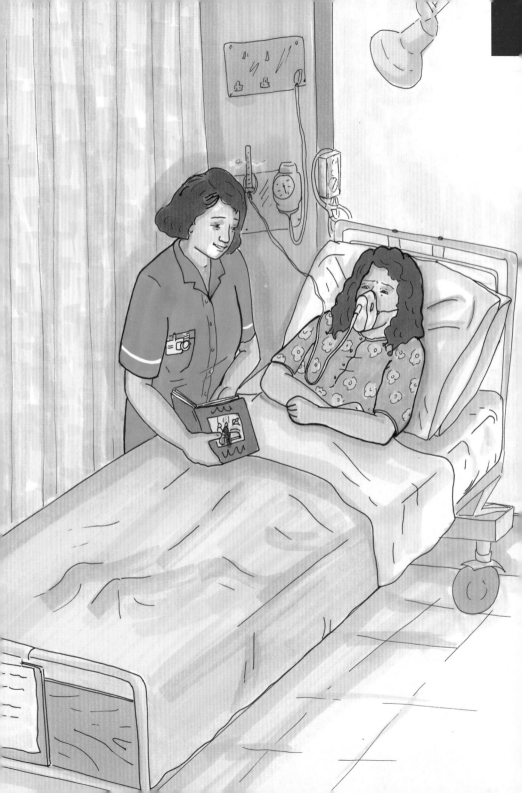

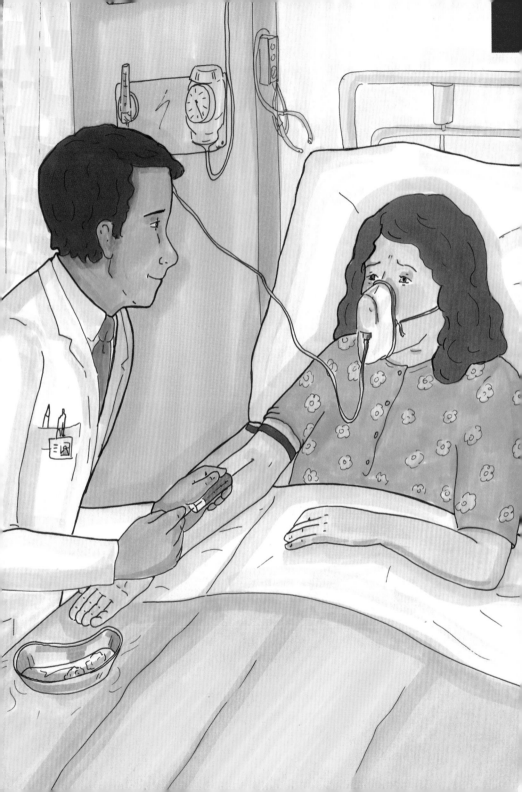

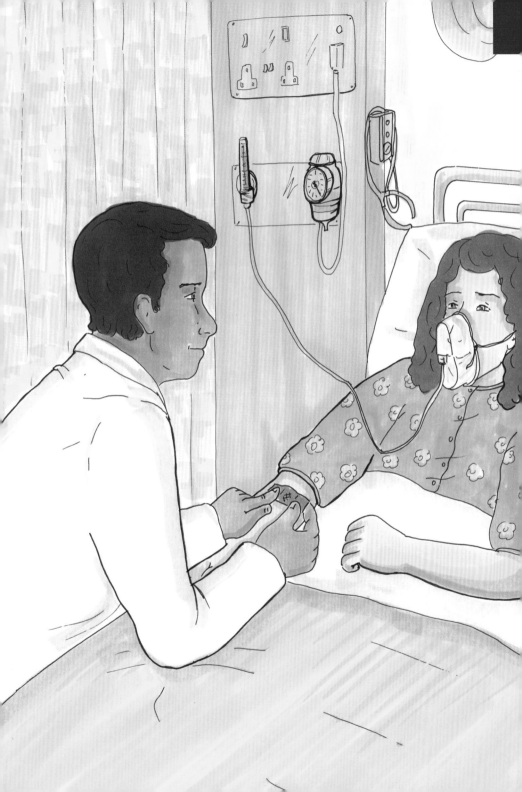

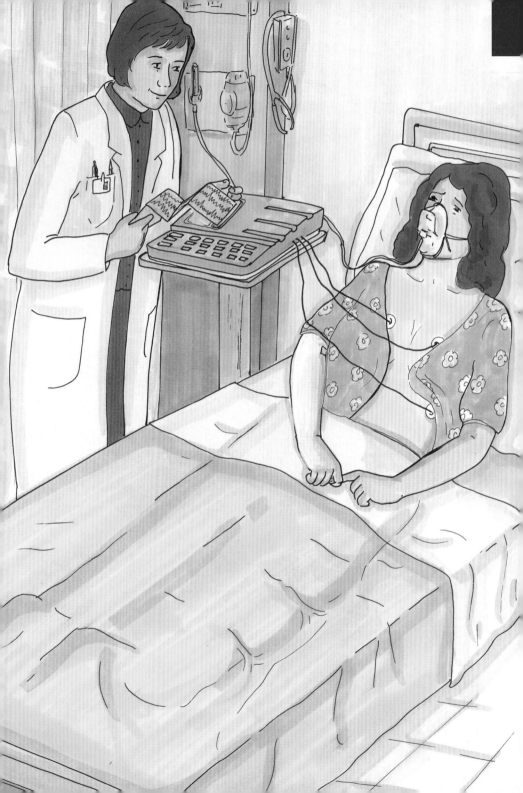

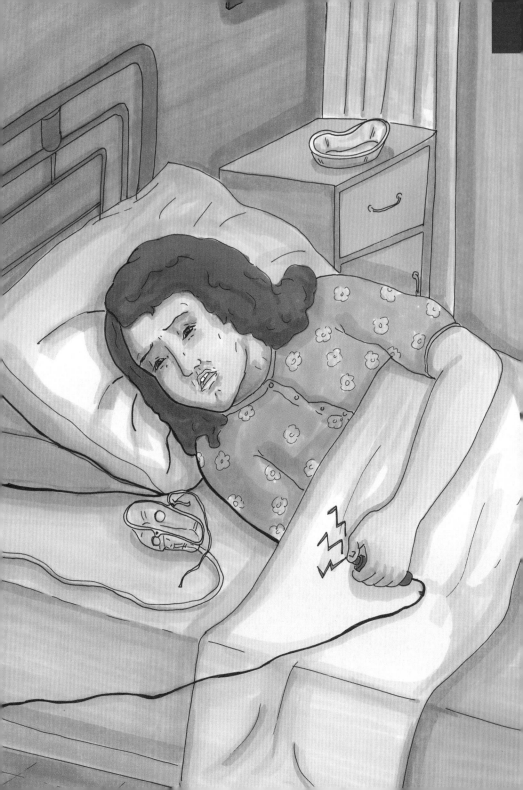

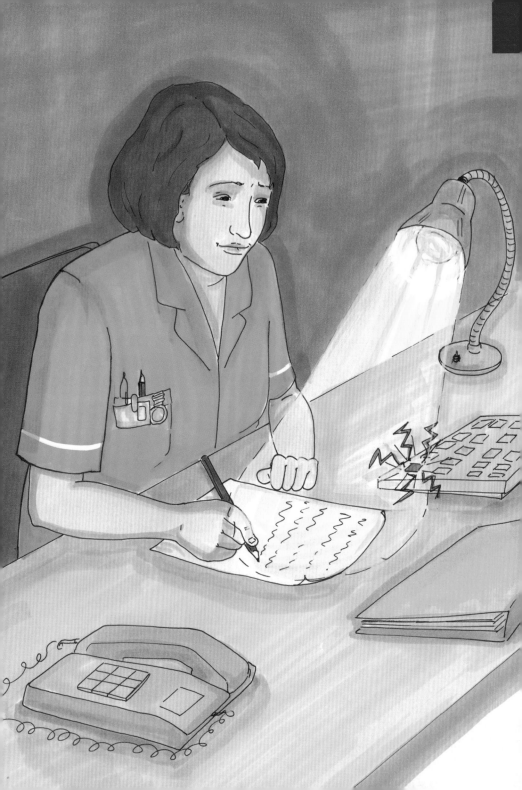

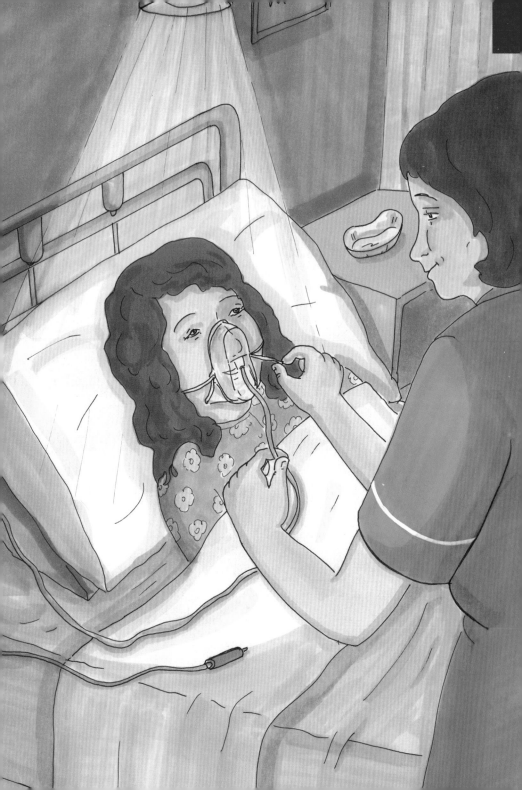

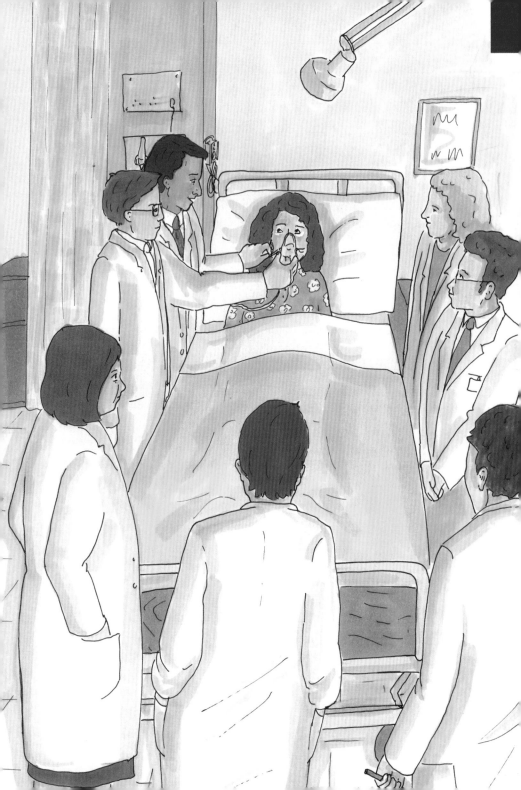

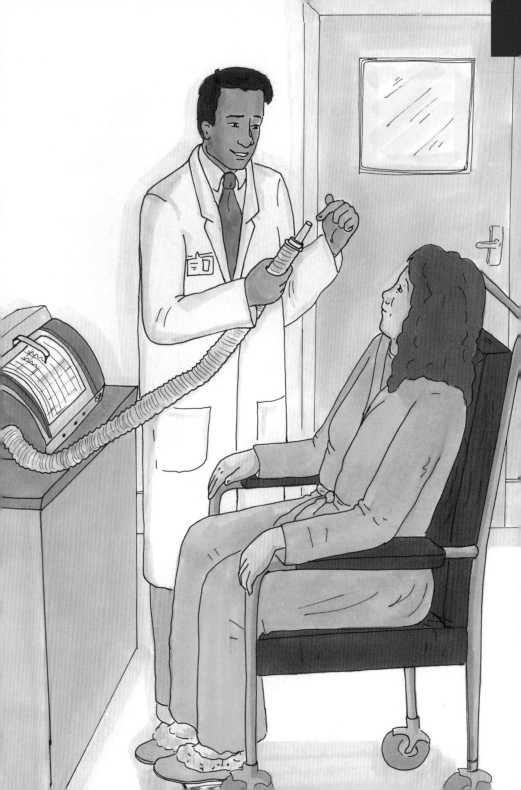

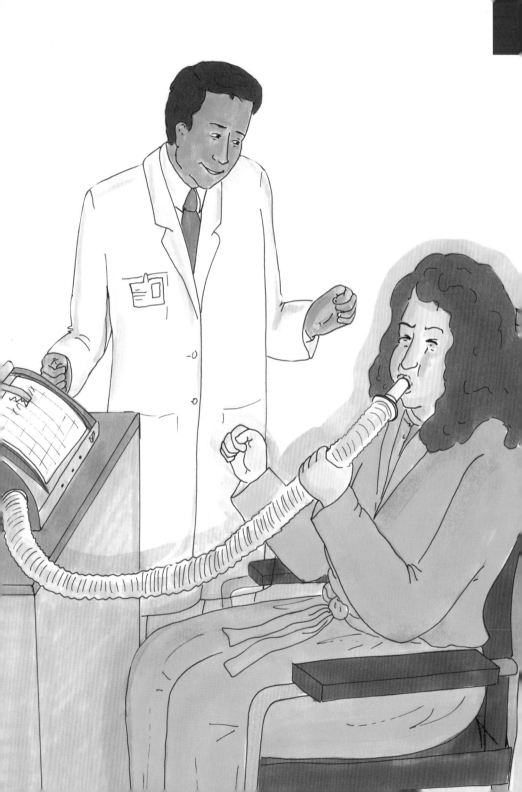

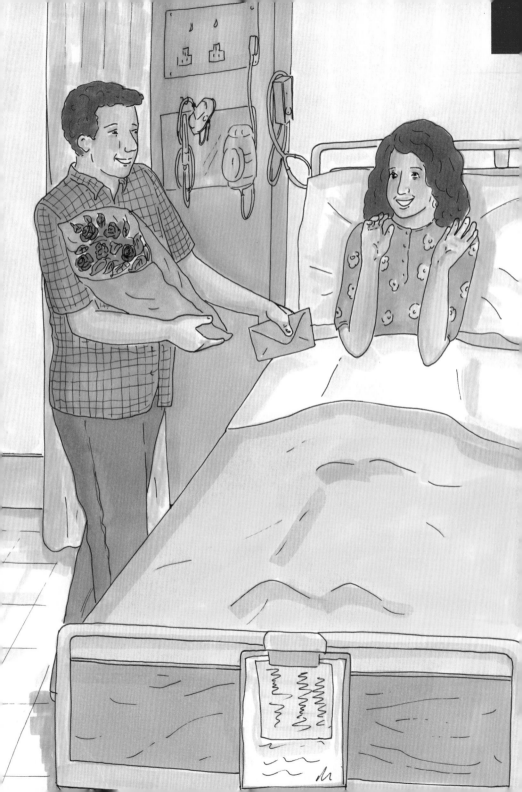

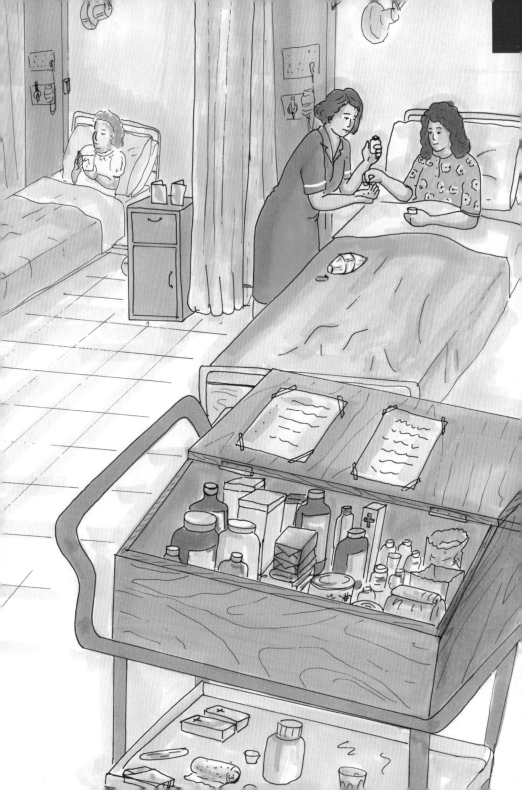

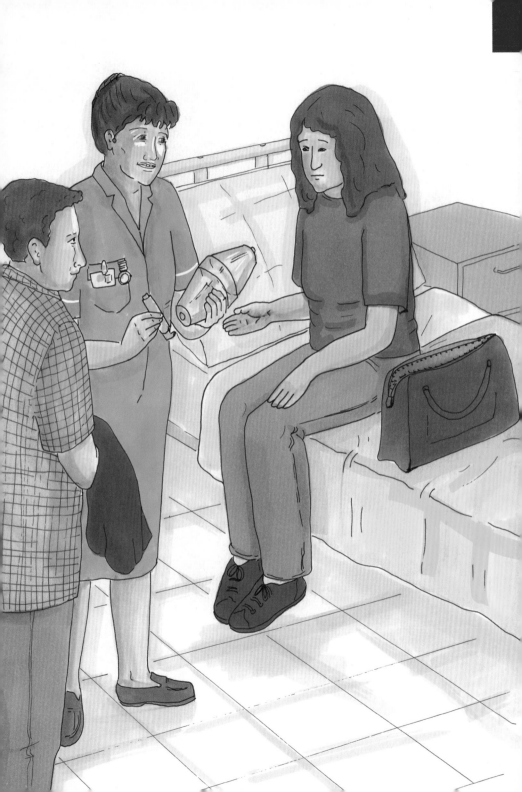

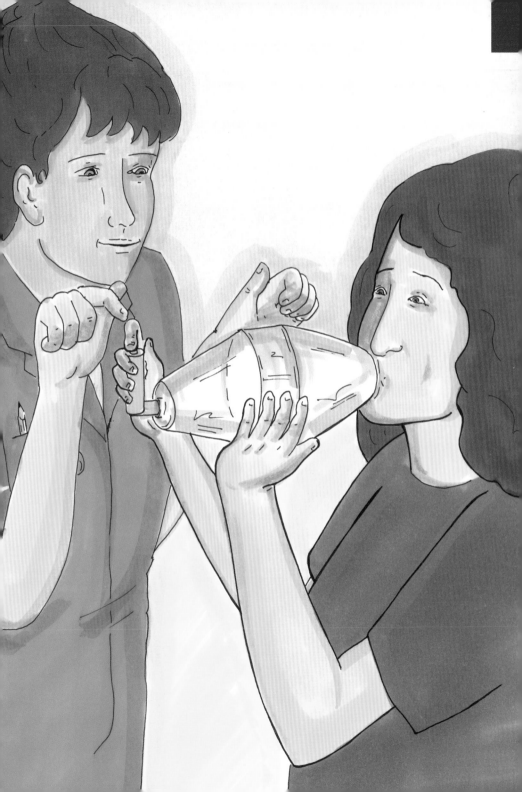

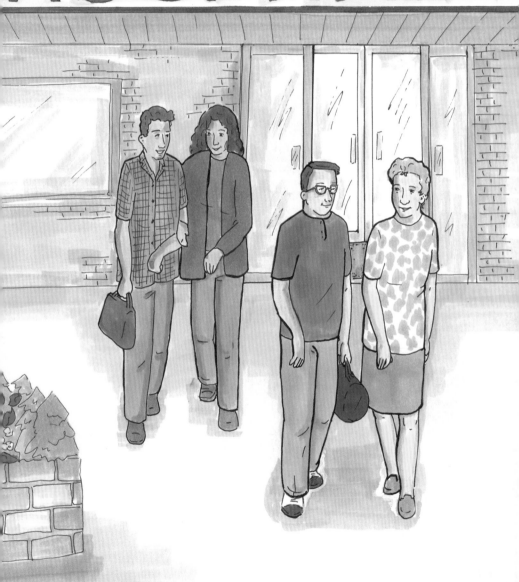

Storyline

The following words are provided for readers and supporters who want some ideas about one possible story. Most readers make their own story up from the pictures.

Martin goes into hospital

1. Martin goes into hospital. His mum is with him.

2. Martin asks the receptionist for help. She tells him where to go.

3. A nurse welcomes him to the ward. Martin is staying there.

4. Another nurse says: "This is your bed."

5. Martin puts on his pyjamas. His mum unpacks his bag.

6. The nurse explains things to him.

7. First, the nurse weighs him.

8. The nurse takes his temperature.

9. The nurse checks Martin's blood pressure.

10. The nurse asks Martin to wee into the bottle.

11. Now he shows him some stockings.

12. He helps Martin pull the stockings on. They feel uncomfortable.

13. Martin climbs into bed.

14. The doctor comes to ask Martin some questions. His mum is there to help if Martin needs her.

15. The doctor pulls the curtain round the bed. She asks Martin to undo his pyjama jacket. She wants to examine his tummy.

16. The doctor explains something to Martin. She tells him he needs to have an operation.

17. Martin decides to say yes to the operation. He signs a consent form.

18. He says goodbye to his mum.

19. The porter takes him somewhere in a wheelchair.

20. He has an x-ray.

21. The radiographer looks at the x-ray.

22. The nurse helps Martin to put on a special gown. He gets ready for his operation.

23. Now he is taken to the operating theatre.

24. The anaesthetist puts a needle into Martin's hand. She uses the needle to give him some medicine. He goes to sleep for his operation.

25. Martin has his operation.

26. Martin wakes up in the recovery room.

27. The nurse takes the needle out of his hand.

28. Martin reads in bed.

29. It's visiting time! His mum comes to see him.

30. The doctor asks Martin how he feels now.

31. The therapist helps Martin to walk.

32. He has his stitches out.

33. Martin is better. He goes home now.

Mary is taken to the emergency department

34. An ambulance arrives at the hospital.

35. Mary is very ill. She lies on a trolley. Her boyfriend is with her.

36. Mary waits to see the doctor.

37. The doctor listens to Mary's chest.

38. The doctor asks Mary some questions. He gives her a nebuliser. This helps her to breathe.

39. The porter takes Mary to the ward. Her boyfriend goes with her too.

40. The nurse explains something to Mary.

41. The doctor takes some blood from Mary.

42. Now he puts a plaster on her arm.

43. Mary has an ECG (a heart test).

44. Mary's mask falls off. She presses the call button.

45. The nurse's light flashes. Is it an emergency?

46. The nurse helps Mary by putting her oxygen mask back on.

47. Mary's doctor and some other doctors and students do a ward round.

48. The doctor wants her to do a lung function test.

49. Mary breathes into the tube.

50. It's visiting time! Mary's boyfriend brings her some flowers.

51. The nurse gives Mary some medicine.

52. Mary is much better. The nurse gives her some medicine to take home. She needs a spacer.

53. Mary tries the spacer.

54. Mary and Martin both go home.

A guide for supporters

Supporters can be parents or other relatives, friends, paid carers, advocates or health professionals. They can be anybody who knows the patient well and goes to an appointment with them to provide information or care, or to help them speak up for themselves.

This book is designed to support people with learning disabilities, like Martin and Mary, when they go into hospital. It explains what happens, and shows events as common as arriving at the main hospital reception desk, to experiences that may cause embarrassment or pain, like assessments and surgery. The pictures will help the reader understand and communicate about experiences and events in hospital.

In England and Wales, the law (Equality Act 2010) requires health and other services to make reasonable adjustments to the way they work to make it as accessible as possible for disabled people. In practice this can mean anything from reducing waiting times and giving information in a way that people understand, to allowing supporters and carers to remain with someone who needs extra help. If the person has a hospital passport (see page 71), staff should use this to find out about the patient's additional needs, and base their approach on this. This book, *Going into Hospital*, is also a valuable communication tool that can help health care workers meet the legal requirement to adjust their practice, as well as to explore capacity and consent.

This book can also be used beyond the hospital, in education or group work to help people learn about what happens in hospital, and to role play different situations. By giving readers the opportunity to engage with another character and see the world through their eyes, the book provides a safe and involving way to explore new or challenging ideas.

Planned admission

If someone you support is going into hospital for a planned operation or procedure, it may be very helpful to look at the pictures in the book beforehand. This will help them to explore how they feel about going into hospital, and learn about some of the things that may happen. For example, by following the pictures featuring Martin, you could prepare someone for expected events such as having their urine tested, being weighed, having an x-ray or an anaesthetic, recovering from the anaesthetic, or having stitches removed.

When the person you support knows the story well, they can use it to communicate with health care staff themselves, which will give them more control over their hospital experience and can reduce fear greatly.

Supporters can get in contact with hospital staff several weeks before a planned operation, to get information and advice about hospital procedures and routines, and to arrange a pre-admission visit to the ward with the patient. This allows the staff to consider each patient's additional needs and to make any reasonable and necessary adjustments to hospital procedures, so that the person's hospital stay goes as well as possible.

Many hospitals have a learning disability nurse working in them. These are nurses trained just to work with people with learning disabilities, to make sure their care meets their needs while they are in hospital, and to help them get the support they require when they go home. So ask if the hospital has a specialist learning disability nurse and say you would like to meet them.

Emergency admission

Arriving at hospital after an accident or sudden medical emergency can be extremely frightening, especially if there are extra barriers of understanding or communication between the patient and staff. The environment in an emergency department is noisy and hectic, and staff may not have specialist skills in working with people with learning disabilities.

On arrival at the emergency department, the supporter should tell hospital staff if the patient has any additional needs. Any supportive materials, such as a hospital passport, if you have been able to bring one, will make the situation easier. A copy of this picture book kept on the ward will help you, the person you support, and busy hospital staff to communicate effectively about what is going to happen. This will help to lessen anxiety and ensure that staff get reliable consent for the things they need to do.

How to explain some medical words simply

Anaesthetic: Before you go into the operating theatre a doctor called an anaesthetist will come to see you. The anaesthetist will put a needle into your hand which may sting a little. The anaesthetist will give you a special medicine called an anaesthetic through this needle. This medicine will make you go to sleep until the operation is over.

Blood pressure: Your heart pumps blood around your body. A doctor or nurse can find out if your heart is working properly by measuring blood pressure in your arm. This does not hurt. Most people have normal blood pressure, but sometimes it can be too high or too low and the doctor can help get it back to normal.

Blood test: The doctor may want to take some blood to see if it's OK or if the medicine you're taking is working properly. To do this the doctor, nurse or health care assistant will use a needle and some special bottles. The needle pricks your arm and the blood goes in the bottle.

Consent: Before you have any treatment or tests, the doctor or nurse must explain what they want to do and why, and what would happen if you did not have it done. You have to decide if you want that test or treatment and agree to it. If you do not agree then they cannot give you the treatment or test. You may be asked to write your name on a piece of paper to say yes.

Examination: This is when the doctor, nurse or therapist has to do something to you to see how you are, for example listening to your chest as you breathe in and out, or touching where it hurts. You may have to take some clothes off for the doctor, nurse or therapist to see or feel properly.

Injection: An injection is a way of giving medicine through a needle. Injections may be given in the arm, bottom or stomach. They do hurt a little.

Medication (also called **drugs**): When you are unwell the doctor may ask you to take one or more medicines to help you get better. Medicines can be ointments or creams, liquids or syrups, tablets or capsules, drops or sprays. Some have to be breathed in using an inhaler and a spacer, or through a mask.

Oxygen mask: This is a plastic cup that is placed over your mouth and nose. Air or oxygen is blown through it to make it easier for you to breathe. The air may feel a bit cold but it is not painful, and you can breathe normally. Sometimes a smaller plastic cup called a nebuliser is attached to the mask. A special liquid medicine is put in the nebuliser to make it easier for you to breathe.

Recovery room: After you have had your operation you will wake up in another room called the recovery room. You may see lots of machines around you. Some of them will make beeping noises. Don't worry – they are all normal. You may have a mask on your face – this is to help you breathe. You may have a bag with liquid attached to the needle going into your hand. You may have a tube sticking out of where you normally wee from – this is so you don't have to get up to go to the toilet. You may have another tube coming out of the place on your body where the operation was – this is to help the wound to heal. Some of these things will be taken away once you are awake. Some may be there for a few days. Ask the nurse if you are worried about anything.

Stitches: These are pieces of special thread used to close up your operation. Sometimes the stitches dissolve by themselves, but other times the nurse needs to take them out. The nurse will use special scissors to cut the stitches and will pull them out with tweezers. It does not normally hurt to have the stitches out.

Stockings: While you are on the ward you may have to wear special stockings. The nurse will help you to put them on. They may feel funny and a bit tight at first but you will soon get used to them. It is important to wear them as they stop your legs swelling up.

Temperature: The nurse will need to measure how hot you are. This is done by using a special small glass tube called a thermometer. The nurse will put the end of the thermometer either under your tongue or under the top of your arm. It is important not to talk if the thermometer is in your mouth. It does not hurt and only takes a few minutes to do.

Theatre: This is the room where you will be taken to have your operation. On the day of your operation (and sometimes the night before) you will not be allowed to eat or drink. You will have to change into a special gown – the nurse will help you do this, and will go with you to the theatre.

Urine test: The nurse may ask you to go to the toilet and wee into a jug, a special bottle or a small pot. This is so that your wee (also called **urine**) can be tested. This can be a bit embarrassing.

X-ray: This is a type of photograph which can see the bones and air inside your body. The photograph is taken by a person called a radiographer. For some x-rays you will have to stand up, and for others you will have to sit or lie down. The radiographer will help you get in the right position and tell you what to do. When the photograph is taken you will be asked to keep very still or, if it is a picture of your chest, you may be asked to take a big breath in.

A guide for hospital staff

This book is designed to help patients with additional needs, such as communication or learning disabilities, to understand and communicate about what is happening when they go into hospital.

Many people will find it helpful to use these pictures to support the information that you give. The pictures are in a story sequence and can either be used before attending hospital by way of preparation or while in the hospital. This will help the patient to ask appropriate questions, and help you know how much your patient understands so that you can obtain informed and reliable consent.

Making reasonable adjustments

The Equality Act 2010 requires services to make 'reasonable adjustments' to support all people with protected characteristics to make full use of their service. This includes people with learning disabilities. The Act also specifies that services must anticipate and plan for the needs of people with protected characteristics when considering what adjustments to make, rather than simply reacting to needs as they are presented.

Caring for patients who have learning disabilities can take time. Some people may find it very difficult to be kept waiting. They may need a double appointment to assess their needs or more than one appointment to familiarise themselves with a proposed procedure beforehand. They may need their carer or supporter to be with them in the anaesthetic room and the recovery room before and after a surgical procedure. Other examples of reasonable adjustments include:

- providing relevant information in a form that the patient understands, such as the pictures in this book

- changing the physical environment, for example by lowering lighting levels, or using a quiet room with fewer distractions and stresses

- offering the first or last appointment to minimise their time in the waiting room

- providing a higher staffing level to meet the patient's additional needs

If hospital staff are worried about meeting the needs of patients with learning disabilities, they can contact the specialist learning disability nurse, if the hospital has one, or their local Community Learning Disability Team (CLDT). If a patient is known to the CLDT, the team can often provide advice and assistance during the patient's hospital stay and at times of admission and discharge. They can also sometimes provide more general training to hospital staff on how to meet the needs of patients with learning disabilities.

Supporters

Some people will come to hospital with a family member, advocate or support worker whose role it is to support their attendance and assist communication. If the patient's supporter knows them well, they can be a vital source of information. Do check how long the supporter has known the patient, and whether there is anyone else, such as a family carer, who needs to be consulted. The patient often relies on their supporter to help describe symptoms or their overall health picture. Sometimes the patient will require a carer or personal assistant to stay with them all the time they are in hospital, and this should be allowed and supported by hospital staff. However, in the UK supporters are not there to do skilled nursing tasks or to substitute for hospital staff.

It is also important to remember not to rely just on the supporter and expect them to speak for the patient, but to speak directly to the patient, and as much as possible take the time and effort to establish a good, respectful and relaxed rapport with them. The supporter's knowledge can then be used to supplement the patient's own report.

Communication

Good communication with the patient, and with their supporter, is crucial to good safe treatment and care. Too often, misunderstandings of a patient's condition or behaviour have led to health care professionals missing a crucial diagnosis or refusing to treat a patient, and patients suffering unnecessarily and even dying as a result. Taking the time and using effective communication tools to explore the patient's physical symptoms and their feelings in a way that is sensitive and appropriate to them will help hospital staff to make the correct diagnosis and keep the patient safe.

Many people with learning disabilities use signs or symbols (e.g. Makaton) instead of speech or to support speech. The patient's supporter should be able to interpret whatever communication system the patient uses. Hospital staff can also be creative and use whatever additional tools work best, for example pictures, posters or sample objects. This book is an example of a how you can support your verbal communication with the patient. Remember that many people with learning disabilities do find pictures easier to understand than words.

The person's non-verbal behaviour is also often a key way that they will communicate their physical and emotional state. This sort of communication may not follow expected patterns, so it is important to check with the patient and with their supporter and to get as much information as you can about what their particular non-verbal communication might mean. For example, subtle changes in the way a person moves their body, as well as more noticeable behaviour changes, such as banging their head against a hard surface, may indicate that a person is in pain.

Hospital passports

Many people with learning disabilities use a document called a hospital passport. These documents can be filled in in advance, and are designed to give hospital staff much of the information they need to give good, safe, person-centred care to the patient.

There is no fixed format for a hospital passport, but most use a 'traffic light' system to give information in an ordered way, with the most critical first.

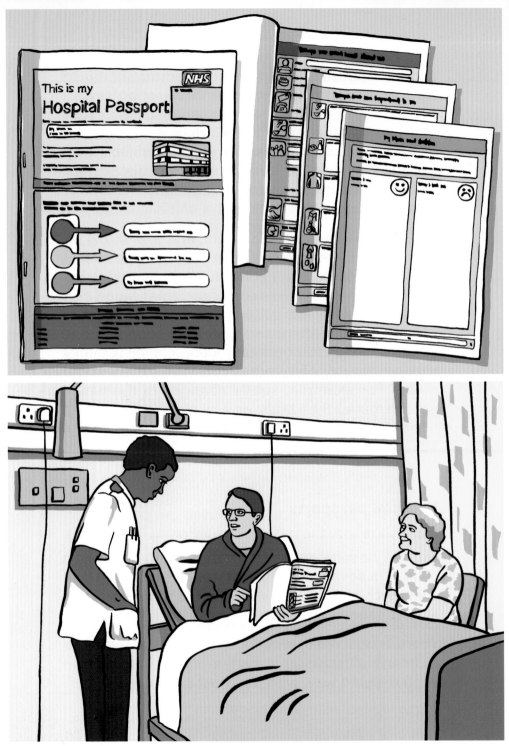

Illustrations by Lucy Bergonzi © Books Beyond Words, 2015.

In the example opposite, the red pages show "things you must know about me", such as important health information, next of kin and so on; the yellow pages show "things that are important to me", such as the patient's ways of communicating, eating and toileting; and the green page shows "my likes and dislikes", for example familiar or favourite activities or topics of conversation.

In a busy emergency department, and depending on the condition the patient is in, it may not be possible or necessary to look at more than the first one or two sections. For a planned admission it will be helpful for a key staff member, such as the 'named nurse', to sit down with the patient and supporter to look at the passport together, and to record it in the patient's notes to ensure consistent care.

The picture at the bottom of the page opposite shows Martin sharing his hospital passport with the nurse when he is admitted to hospital. His mum is there to help if she is needed. Many patients with learning disabilities will not be able to explain things themselves, and a carer or support worker will be the person who introduces the passport. In every situation, the patient should be as involved as possible in discussing their care.

Consent

This book emphasises the importance of consent and provides pictures that may help to clarify the choices open to the patient.

According to the Mental Capacity Act (2005) for the patient's consent to be valid, the patient must be able to:

- understand the information relevant to the decision

- retain the information long enough to make the decision

- use or weigh up the information

- communicate their decision.

Information relevant to the decision must be provided in a form that the patient can understand. This means explaining what is involved in simple terms and short sentences, and being willing to repeat or reword explanations.

The pictures in this book may help you to explain something and to check how much your patient has understood. The person may be able to repeat the information to you in their own words or they may show that they understand and consent by their non-verbal communication or behaviour, for example by rolling up their sleeve for a blood test.

In the first instance you should assume that the patient has capacity to make a decision, and use all available tools to help them demonstrate that capacity. If the patient is not able to give informed consent, even with maximal support, then the clinical decision maker should:

- consider whether the decision can be delayed if the person is expected to regain capacity

- act in the best interests of the person

- consider holding a Best Interest meeting under the Mental Capacity Act

- always use the less restrictive option

- encourage participation in the decision

- consult all relevant people

- if the person has no relatives, consider a referral to an Independent Mental Capacity Advocate (IMCA).

Hospital staff should remember that mental capacity is time-, location- and decision-specific, and just because a patient is unable to make a particular decision, it does not mean they lack capacity to consent to other types of medical treatment, or to make decisions in other areas of their life.

A short video showing how to obtain informed consent for a blood test is available at: www.youtube.com/watch?v=rJS6ahXKbik.

Key points in working with patients with learning disabilities

- Be respectful. Don't make assumptions about a person's quality of life. Treat the patient in a way that is appropriate to their chronological age.

- Respect confidentiality, as for any other patient.

- Always communicate with the patient directly. If a person does not use verbal language to communicate, use pictures like the ones in this book, photos, symbols, sign etc. to engage with them.

- Assess people's health and wellbeing so that any changes in behaviour that may signify changes in condition or an illness are not attributed to their learning disability.

- Pay close attention to non-verbal communication, for example sounds, body positions, facial gestures and other non-verbal signs that may indicate pain, anxiety, discomfort and understanding.

- Be aware of the physical setting and how you can adjust it to support the patient's access, comfort and safety.

- Read and act upon the patient's hospital passport.

- Understand the issues around gaining consent clearly, and make every effort to gain consent.

- Seek out help from people who know the patient best and engage with family or supporters to help you communicate effectively with them. This may help you get to know the person and understand what is in their best interests if they lack capacity to consent.

- Ensure that the lines of communication with the patient, their family carers, advocates or supporters are clearly established throughout their inpatient journey. Always inform the person's family carers, advocates or supporters when they are moved from one area to another.

- Always liaise with Community Learning Disability Team colleagues and other community clinicians, for example GPs, to support admission and discharge, or if someone with a learning disability does not turn up for an appointment.

Useful resources

Services in the UK

Community Learning Disability Teams (CLDTs)

These are specialist multidisciplinary health teams that support adults with learning disabilities and their families by assessment of their health needs and a range of clinical interventions. The composition of CLDTs varies, but will usually include psychology, psychiatry and nursing with a range of therapeutic specialists such as speech and language therapy, occupational therapy and physiotherapy. Referral to the local CLDT is encouraged for both developmental and therapeutic work. Some are joint health and social work teams and have a social care management role as well.

Social service departments

Social service departments manage and purchase social care, for example, housing and day services for people with learning disabilities.

Mencap

Mencap is a UK charity working with and for people with a learning disability and their parents and carers. The health section on their website provides useful videos, guides and leaflets for professionals, people with learning disabilities, their families and supporters. Mencap has a lot of local knowledge, and a network of connections nationwide. This means that they can link you up with organisations or services in your area that can help. They also run an information and advice helpline that offers free, confidential and

independent information and advice on virtually any subject to do with learning disability.
www.mencap.org.uk
Helpline: 0808 808 1111

Office of the Public Guardian
Supports the Public Guardian in the registration of Enduring Powers of Attorney (EPA) and Lasting Powers of Attorney (LPA), and the supervision of deputies appointed by the Court of Protection. It also helps attorneys and deputies to carry out their duties, and protects people who lack the mental capacity to make decisions for themselves.
www.justice.gov.uk/about/opg

Written materials available on the internet

Healthcare for All: Independant Inquiry into Access to Healthcare for People with Learning Disabilities, by Sir Jonathan Michael (2008). The Michael Report is a comprehensive report into the health inequalities experienced by people with learning disabilities. It makes a number of recommendations including annual health checks and better support for people with learning disabilities in hospital.
http://webarchive.nationalarchives.gov.uk/20130107105354/http:/www.dh.gov.uk/prod_consum_dh/groups/dh_digitalassets/@dh/@en/documents/digitalasset/dh_106126.pdf

Understanding Intellectual Disability and Health. A learning resource for practitioners and students about the health and social care needs of people with learning disabilities.
www.intellectualdisability.info/

Easy Health
A website with easy-to-understand information about staying healthy and getting help with your health. Most resources are free to download, including a number of example hospital passports.
www.easyhealth.org.uk

Meeting needs and reducing distress. An **NHS Protect** project output providing guidance on the prevention and management of clinically related challenging behaviour in NHS settings. The website offers guidance documents, case studies, training videos and other resources and tools that will be useful for health care professionals.
www.reducingdistress.co.uk/reducingdistress/

Working together: easy steps to improving how people with a learning disability are supported when in hospital. Produced by Hft (formerly Home Farm Trust), a national charity providing services for people with learning disabilities, this free booklet offers guidance for hospitals, families and paid support staff about what they can each do to help ensure that people with learning disabilities get the support that is right for them and the most effective treatment during their hospital stay.
www.hft.org.uk/Supporting-people/family-carers/Resources/Health-resources/

Everybody's life has worth – Getting it right in hospital for people with an intellectual disability and reducing clinical risks, by Jim Blair. An article detailing various ways of reducing the risk of diagnostic overshadowing and poor treatment by using good quality communication tools and making effective

adjustments to nursing practice, including reliable assessments of capacity.
http://cri.sagepub.com/content/19/3/58.full.pdf

Asthma UK has produced a number of easy read materials to help people better understand and manage their condition. Resources are free to download.
www.asthma.org.uk/downloads

Related titles in the Books Beyond Words series

Going to the Doctor (1996) by Sheila Hollins, Jane Bernal and Matthew Gregory, illustrated by Beth Webb. This book illustrates a variety of experiences which may occur during a visit to the GP. These include meeting the doctor, having one's ears syringed, a physical examination, a blood test, a blood pressure check and getting a prescription.

Going to Out-Patients (2009, 2nd edition) by Sheila Hollins, Jane Bernal and Matthew Gregory, illustrated by Denise Redmond. This book explains what happens in out-patient departments, covering tests such as ultrasound, x-ray and hearing tests. Feelings, information and consent to treatment are addressed.

Ann has Dementia (2012) by Sheila Hollins, Noëlle Blackman and Ruth Eley, illustrated by Lisa Kopper. Ann is diagnosed with dementia. We see her GP and her supporter caring for Ann in the early days of her dementia until she becomes so confused that she has to move into residential care.

Getting on with Cancer (2002) by Veronica Donaghey, Jane Bernal, Irene Tuffrey-Wijne and Sheila Hollins, illustrated by Beth Webb. This book tells the story of Veronica who has various treatments for cancer, including radiotherapy, chemotherapy and surgery. It deals honestly with the unpleasant side of treatment and ends on a positive note.

Getting on with Epilepsy (2014, 2nd edition) by Sheila Hollins, Jane Bernal and Alice Thacker, illustrated by

Lisa Kopper. This book illustrates experiences that are worrying for people with epilepsy, like having seizures in public, going to the doctor, having a brain scan, EEG or blood test, and taking daily medication. Activities such as safe drinking, swimming and cooking are covered, showing that it is possible to enjoy an active and independent life with epilepsy.

Looking After My Heart (2005) by Sheila Hollins, Francesco Cappuccio and Paul Adeline, illustrated by Lisa Kopper. Jane likes to smoke, drink alcohol and eat party food. Only after she has a heart attack and is taken to hospital, does she begin to look after herself better. She is given medication and advice on healthy eating to prevent further heart disease and, in time, makes a full recovery.

Authors

Sheila Hollins is Emeritus Professor of Psychiatry of Disability at St George's, University of London, and sits in the House of Lords. She is a past President of the Royal College of Psychiatrists and of the BMA. She is founding editor of Books Beyond Words and Executive Chair of Beyond Words, and a family carer for her son who has a learning disability.

Angie Avis was Superintendent Physiotherapist in Learning Disabilities in South West London.

Samantha Cheverton was a Senior Nursing Sister at St George's Hospital.

Jim Blair is Consultant Nurse, Learning Disabilities, at Great Ormond Street Hospital. He is also Associate Professor of Intellectual Disabilities at Kingston and St George's Universities, and Health Advisor at the British Institute of Learning Disabilities.

Denise Redmond, the artist, previously worked at St George's University of London.

Acknowledgments

We are grateful to many people who gave their time most generously to help us, in particular: Dr Jane Bernal, Anna Cawdery, Laraine Rawford, Veronica Donaghey, Dorothea Duncan, Matthew Gregory, Nigel Hollins, Dr Bernard Liban, Jane Penny, Wendy Perez, Dr Charlotte Rayner.

Thanks also to the staff and Women's Group at Blakes and Link Employment Agency (Hammersmith & Fulham Social Services) and the nursing staff on Amyand Ward, St George's Hospital.

This edition of *Going into Hospital* has been made possible by a generous grant from the British Medical Association.

Beyond Words: publications and training

Books Beyond Words are stories for anyone who finds pictures easier than words. A list of all Beyond Words publications, including print and eBook versions of Books Beyond Words titles, and where to buy them, can be found on our website:

www.booksbeyondwords.co.uk

Workshops for family carers, support workers and professionals about using Books Beyond Words are provided regularly in London, or can be arranged in other localities on request. Self-advocates are welcome. For information about forthcoming workshops see our website or contact us:

email: admin@booksbeyondwords.co.uk

Video clips showing our books being read are also on our website and YouTube channel: www.youtube.com/user/booksbeyondwords and on our DVD, *How to Use Books Beyond Words*.

How to read this book

There is no right or wrong way to read this book. Remember it is not necessary to be able to read the words.

1. Some people are not used to reading books. Start at the beginning and read the story in each picture. Encourage the reader to hold the book themselves and to turn the pages at their own pace.

2. Whether you are reading the book with one person or with a group, encourage them to tell the story in their own words. You will discover what each person thinks is happening, what they already know, and how they feel. You may think something different is happening in the pictures yourself, but that doesn't matter. Wait to see if their ideas change as the story develops. Don't challenge the reader(s) or suggest their ideas are wrong.

3. Some pictures may be more difficult to understand. It can help to prompt the people you are supporting, for example:

- Who do you think that is?
- What is happening?
- What is he or she doing now?
- How is he or she feeling?
- Do you feel like that? Has it happened to you/ your friend/ your family?

4. You don't have to read the whole book in one sitting. Allow people enough time to follow the pictures at their own pace.

5. Some people will not be able to follow the story, but they may be able to understand some of the pictures. Stay a little longer with the pictures that interest them.